Weaving the Sound
of Heart

Weaving the Sound of Heart

Solving the Agonies with Healing Energy: Hado Power

Toyoko MATSUZAKI
Translated by Natsumi KUROKI

iUniverse, Inc.
New York Lincoln Shanghai

Weaving the Sound of Heart
Solving the Agonies with Healing Energy: Hado Power

iUniverse, Inc.

For information address:
iUniverse, Inc.
2021 Pine Lake Road, Suite 100
Lincoln, NE 68512
www.iuniverse.com

ISBN: 0-595-29819-2

Printed in the United States of America

CONTENTS

PREFACE

WEAVING THE SOUND OF HEART

Human hearts are like fabrics. The intricate warps and wefts are tangled with unseen "threads."

I sense these unseen threads and I can disentangle them gently so that people can find their peace of mind and their happiness again. I believe this is my special calling.

"I am so miserable now. I am suffering a lot. Please help me." A lot of people suffering deep agonies come to see me: troubles in relationships, husband's unemployment, divorce, accidents, serious illness, domestic violence and so on.

First, I ask my clients to relax and calm down; then I sense the "*hado*" (Note: *"hado"* literally means wave motion in Japanese. Often used as *ki*** or *ki* energy in the spiritual literature. "*Ki*" means the same as *Qi* or *Chi* in Chinese: 'Life force energy') of the sound from them. Using my clairvoyant power, I visualize the true figure of their problems and sufferings. Finally I advise them with all my heart how to cope with the sufferings so that they can solve their difficult problems.

We face many kinds of problems as long as we live; there are many ways to solve them as we disentangle the threads.

Nothing can be solved if you worry all by yourself. Keep firmly in your mind that the first step towards happiness is to have the courage to ask for advice for your problems.

I have a special gift from God to see through the bottom of the heart by sensing the sound and the *hado* released from a person's five senses such as the way they speak, breath and walk.

I wrote this booklet because I felt compelled to let people know about the examples of how I advised and solved my clients' problems.

I would appreciate it if you could take time to read this booklet. It would be my great honor if anyone could break the spells of ill fortune and suffering by reading this book.

MESSAGE FROM THE AUTHOR

When you are sick or feel pain in your body,

Put your hand on the affected area, and

Visualize me.

You will get better.

When you need to change your life,

Or feel that you never find a gleam of hope,

Visualize me.

You will find a way.

I imprinted in this booklet my healing energy ~ the *hado* power,

It will give you power

To make your life better.

STRANGE DREAMS

Summer, 16 years old. I had a strange dream when I dozed off one morning.

A beautiful angel got off from a cow carriage descended from heaven, and she reached out her arms to me.

In awe, I touched her hands.

"You shall go into music. Live your life valuing the compassion which you shall have by listening to the *hado* of music."

One month later, she appeared in my dream again.

"If you follow what I told you, you shall understand people's hearts."

If this happened to a 16-year-old girl of today, she would make fun of it, saying, "No Kidding." Honestly speaking, I was half in doubt but for some reason I decided to follow the words of the angel.

From then on, I studied vocal seriously, studying at *Musashino Academia Musicae College* in Tokyo. After graduating from the College, while I put my heart and soul into music, one day suddenly I could see through people's hearts clearly.

Good fortunes and ill fortunes. Life has various kinds of dramas. Everyone equally has the opportunity to know themselves deeply.

You don't have to suffer all by yourself. Why don't you contact me if you want to broaden your world?

1. VIEWING THE *HADO*

A Master Violin

Due to my profession, I often interact with musicians. One of them, a female orchestral musician showed me her proud possession: a violin. I had heard that it was a very famous masterpiece; however, for some reasons, it didn't feel right to me. Something about it bothered me, so I asked her:

"I guess this violin has belonged to many different master musicians. I sense that it picked up many habits from them. Don't you feel this violin turns away from you?"

She looked surprised. "How did you know? I feel exactly that way. I cannot create good sound out of it…. Actually I think I am in trouble." She looked as though she didn't know what to do with the masterpiece.

I caught the *hado* released from the violin just by observing the way she handled it.

"Maybe I shouldn't say this, but just because you cannot create the sound as good as you intended to, you handle the violin roughly without being aware of it. From now on, when you perform, ask the violin to co-operate with you and to create an excellent sound before the performance."

After this incident, she went on a concert tour. After a while, she called me from her travel destination.

"As you advised me, I handled the violin with care and asked it to cooperate with me with all my heart before the performance. And you know, I could play so excellently! Members of orchestra told me I did a good job!"

Her voice was in a cheerful sound as well. Even a masterpiece will turn away from you if you treat it roughly. Please try to communicate with all things.

Singing Heals Atopic Dermatitis

"My daughter is suffering from terrible atopic dermatitis. Is there any way we can treat her?" A mother visited me with her 16 year old daughter. Poor daughter – her neck was festered. Somehow, she gave me a somber impression.

By intuition, "Do you like singing?" I asked the daughter. Her face brightened, and she answered me, "Yes, I love it!"

I was so surprised to hear her voice: she had a strong and beautiful soprano voice. I told the mother to treat her daughter's dermatitis with vocal lessons but she looked doubtful. "Really? Does she have that kind of talent?"

"It is understandable that any parents can miss their children's talent. By listening to her voice, I can clearly see her gift of song. What are you going to do?" I asked.

They went home so that the mother could consult with her husband. The mother and the daughter returned the next day.

The mother stated: "I spoke with my husband. He says, 'What a funny thing Ms. Matsuzaki said. Why don't we dare to leave the matter to her?' Please give my daughter vocal lessons."

So the daughter started the vocal lessons. Soon she showed her exceptional talent and her atopic dermatitis was healed in no time. As she built self-confidence, she started to have better grades at school, and passed the college entrance examination for the singing course in a breeze.

Family environment greatly affects the symptoms of atopic dermatitis; it can be healed by relieving stress. Being too strict about child discipline builds up stress in your children. We all should keep that in mind.

Koto Concert

A Master of *koto* (Japanese Harp) who has a lot of pupils visited me. "I enjoy playing *koto* surrounded by young pupils. A while ago, I had a nightmare: in the dream, I played and played but no sound came out of my *koto*. That made me very nervous. Please flow *ki* energy into me so that I can perform the *koto* without any worries at the upcoming concert."

While I flew the *ki* into her, I tried the clairvoyant power with *hado* that gave me a vision of a gentle flow of a river.

"I see a gentle flow of a river. Don't worry. The concert will be successful." Then she gave a gasp.

"How far you can see through? One of the tunes I play has a motif of 'a gentle flow of a river.' I am surprised."

I guaranteed that the concert would be of success and told her to enjoy playing the koto with confidence but she was not yet convinced. "Would you come and flow *ki* energy into me before the concert?"

As promised, I visited her rehearsal hall and flew *ki* energy into her and her instrument. While I observed their lessons, her pupils started to say, "Sounds much better." "I think the sound has been improved." I had the same impression too.

Of course, the sound wouldn't be improved only by flowing *ki*, but I assume that the Master braced herself for playing koto by receiving my *ki* that improved her concentration level.

Furthermore, her self-confidence played the larger part as well, believing everything would be just fine because she received the *ki* energy.

Sometimes you need a refresher for lessons. It is important to approach everything with pure and renewed spirit.

A Young Man of Withdrawal

One of my friends asked me for a consultation concerning her relative. He was a 25 year old man in *Ishigaki* Island and hadn't gotten out of bed for three months. Relatives said he was not sick. He was a very famous dutiful son in the neighborhood. Why had this happened? His mother called her sister, who is my friend, worried.

I sent the *hado* power to the dutiful son in *Ishigaki* Island. I saw a vision of the neighboring landscape. I tried to visualize him in a bed, to my surprise, I saw a tail coming out from his hip.

I kept on sending the *hado* power. Finally it revealed the real figure. It was a turtle. I knew 'This was it!' so I advised my friend, "Call your sister in *Ishigaki* Island and look for a turtle in her house."

The sister called my friend back within ten minutes. "There is a stuffed turtle in a closet." I told her: "Please take the turtle out from there."

I sent the *hado* power to the stuffed turtle. After a brief interval, the turtle went back into the ocean with joy. At the same time, she called me back with excitement.

"My son just got up from the bed and started to wash his face. I looked at him in wonder – and he came to me and said, 'Mother, I am hungry. Can you cook something for me?' so I served him in surprise and he ate everything with relish."

I heard that he went back into a normal life thereafter. I think that the spirit of turtle cursed the kind son for help. *Hado* power has nothing to do with the distance.

Please contact me if you are in trouble.

New York

Four to five years ago, all of a sudden, I started to feel, "I want to go to New York! I have to go to New York!" This feeling was so strong, and it lingered in my mind and heart all the time. People asked me "why New York?" but I had no idea why I felt that way.

Before long, I heard the news of terrifying September 11th.

I visited New York in 2003 to have *hado* sessions with my clients. When I looked towards the south from windows of the hotel I stayed in midtown, and when I cruised down the Hudson River, I felt tightness in my chest and couldn't stop crying for no reasons. I learned that was where the twin towers had been once located.

Usually I don't remember people's name or things long since I meet so many people every day for counseling. However, just sometimes, when I meet particular person or face the particular things, I started to feel uneasy about them and my anxiety stays in my heart. I don't know why but something bad always happens to them afterwards.

There are so many people in New York. These people are releasing positive energy with full of hopes and lives. On the other hand, I felt the negative energies working in people. I might pick up those negative energies without realizing it when I felt strong about New York years ago.

2. VISUALIZATION WITH CLAIRVOYANT POWER

What Business Cards Would Tell You

"Recently I am often cheated by business partners," said a president of a medium-sized company with a gloomy expression. He held out some twenty business cards to me. "They are all important business partners. Please see through them with your clairvoyant power."

I put the business cards on the table and tried the visualization one by one. "I see this person is black-hearted. I wonder what this blackness means…. Will he try to cheat you or….."

Unfortunately, the president had already been cheated. The partner had already been deported but the president kept his business card hoping to collect the debt as it was a huge amount of money.

The next business card made me feel uneasy. "I see the blackness over his legs. Tell this person to be careful." Unfortunately, I later heard that this person had a car accident and injured his legs three months later.

With the third business card, I saw the blackness over a man's mouth, but there was a light within. "He has a big mouth. Not many people trust him but he'll bring you a big business opportunity in near future. If you could be in a leading position, he'd bring you big money."

The president looked half in doubt but somehow he knew what I was trying to tell him. I sensed his "*orion*" (literally means 'waving the sound') *hado* with joy.

As I described, the visualization with *hado* power is able to tell me the person's characteristics and behavior with accuracy. I can also sense the person's heart in front of me by catching the *onion hado* released from them.

I acquired this power though my long music career. Remember, every-body has psychic powers.

Becoming a Buddhist Monk

There is the story of a corporate employee working for a gravestone company in Wakayama Prefecture. He was laid off and came to me for advice for setting up a new gravestone store. He was a short, round-faced, young-looking man, forty years old.

"Would this shop be successful?" He asked.

Suddenly, one Buddhist temple came to my mind. The temple is located along the side of the road I usually drive, and for some reasons, it seems to me to be shining all the time.

I wrote down the name and the map to the temple and gave it to him. "I don't know anybody at this temple but go seek counsel with the resident priest for the new business. I visualize the priest and you cleaning the tem-ple with delight." [Note: cleaning the temple is a part of trainings to become a monk.]

I guess because he had nothing to lose after the layoff, he visited the temple immediately. He spoke to the priest about his business plan with his whole heart, and the priest was willing to offer his advice.

While preparing for the opening of the gravestone shop, he kept on vis-iting the priest. One day the priest said to him:

"There's another temple with which I am associated. From what I can tell, you would be a great resident priest. I'd recommend you to perform the ascentic training seriously to become a Buddhist monk. If you do, I'd take care of all the living expenses until you accomplish this."

"There was no one who thought of me as deeply as the priest." The words of the priest touched this forty year old man's heart deeply.

"I will go with you for the rest of my life, priest."

By leaps and bounds, everything goes very smoothly. Both his job and the ascentic training are going well. He is satisfied with his fulfilling life. Sometimes you can find a chance right under your nose.

PhD Thesis

I have a male best friend who calls me "Boss." He came to seek advice about his PhD thesis. I tried the clairvoyant power with *hado* in front of him. I saw a solid lock attached to an old treasure box. It unlocked with a clang.

"Your theme is about a historical issue." "How did you know?" He said he was studying the period when cows were introduced to Japan. "It sounds interesting. I see everything goes well. Do your best," I advised him.

One year later he contacted me again. He had submitted his thesis to his professor but there was no news after three months of authorization period. "Boss, what's going on?" he asked. He looked worried.

I tried the clairvoyant power again. I saw the professor really liked the thesis, reading it over and over again. "Don't worry. The professor seemed to think very highly of your thesis. Wait a little longer at ease. I'm sure you will receive good news soon."

A few days later, his thesis was returned to him with the highest mark. He told the professor, "I thought I couldn't make it this time because it took so long." "Sorry, I couldn't get back to you sooner. The thesis was so excellent that I was absorbed in reading it." The professor said.

My friend came to report this success delightedly. He thanked me so many times.

"I'll visualize what is to come," I said.

I saw a large ship sailing into the ocean. "Your thesis will be highly thought of overseas, too. Keep on working hard."

After this, he went up the ladder of success. I heard that his thesis is referenced in German medical books.

Desk Layout

An owner of a middle-sized-company came to seek my counsel.

"I brought a desk layout of my company. Would you take a look at it?" he asked.

I saw a light shining from one desk. "Well, whose desk is this? I think the person who sits here has so much potential; he may still be young, but leave a project to him."

Then I saw one desk totally in black. I felt extremely uneasy about it, so I pointed the desk and asked;

"What kind of job this person does?"

He looked so upset. "Well, that desk belongs to one of my sales staff."

"I feel so uneasy about this desk…I strongly recommend you to investigate this person as soon as possible. I have a feeling the person is doing something behind you."

The owner left in a hurry. I sincerely hoped that my advice made difference on his company.

Few years later, when I almost forgot my advice gave to this company owner, I read an article of his company in the newspaper. It says that the person in charge of the sales stole huge amount of money from his company and got arrested. I felt so bad because the owner didn't do anything although he had my advice previously.

After this incident, I had a chance to talk to him in private. He told me that he knew my advice was right deep in his heart but he couldn't do anything because he was dating that person and too scared to find out the truth.

Director's Bad Fortune

"Would you please take a look at this photograph?"

A female office worker came to see me for my advice. She showed me a group photo of her office, taken at a New Years' Party. I was so surprised the air in the photo was extremely stagnant. She continued.

"After taking this picture, the entire employee had series of bad luck. I was robbed on the street; two of my colleagues were hospitalized, and so on. Now everyone became scared saying 'who is the next victim?' We are talking that our office is haunted."

"I don't think your office is cursed or haunted. Don't worry about it. I think everybody in the picture happened to be going through bad period. People who have bad luck tend to get together," I explained to her.

I kept on looking at the picture. I felt insecure about one male employee in the photograph.

"He got car accidents, right?"

My client looked so surprised. "How do you know? He had two car accidents after this party although he never had had one past 10 years."

Then I saw one man in his fifties in the photo. Suddenly I felt that I couldn't even stand to see the photograph and returned it back to her.

"Ay, I cannot see this photograph any more. I see the total blackness over this particular person. Who is he?"

"Oh, it's our director. What's wrong with him?" she said.

"Is he the director of your office? Now I see the whole picture. After he came, don't you think the sales of your office went down?"

"Well, everybody in my company says the director doesn't have luck. Right after becoming the director of my office, the economy went down sharply. Yes, indeed, our sales have been down pretty much since he came," she said.

I guess that the director attracted people who happened to have bad luck like a strong magnet.

My client continued, "I hear that he will become a director of another branch office next month."

"Then, I don't have to do anything this time. You will feel the air in your office would be much better soon. You'll soon see the sales go up too."

She looked half in doubt at that time. However, after the director had left her office, no one in the office suffered bad luck any more and the sales went up pretty much.

The company's fortune is greatly affected by the executive's fortune. In another words, the person in the managing position represent the company's destiny.

3. MESSAGE FROM THE PEOPLE WHO PASSED AWAY

Forgiveness

My son was killed in a car accident. He was just sitting in the passenger's seat and killed. However, the one who caused the accident was survived, ironically. After his death, people who loved him suffered a huge loss for a long time. They didn't know what to think of his death or what to do with their sadness.

One of my friends was so closed to him that she kept his photograph in her car. My son was showing his beautiful smile in the photograph all the time.

One day she suddenly felt impotent rage over the loss of my son when she was driving. She totally lost her control; banging the dashboard and screaming:

"Why? Why he had to die? Why not the one who caused the accident? It is him who was supposed to be killed!"

She stumbled upon my son's photograph; my son wasn't smiling any more. Not only that, he turned away from her.

She burst into tears. She clearly understood my son's message; she should not loathe the person who caused the accident because it was an "accident." The person didn't mean to kill him. She apologized to my son's photograph with tears. He started to show his beautiful smile to her again.

After hearing this story from my friend, I couldn't stop crying and I promised to my son that I would treat the person who caused the accident as if he were my real son. Since my son was such a broad-minded man, I knew that not only he had forgiven the person, but also he worried the person because he felt terrible guilt over what he had done to my son.

I think my son sent us a very important message. When the loved one is killed in an accident, the bereaved family and friends shouldn't loathe the person who caused it as long as the person takes the responsibility. Your loved one has already forgiven the person in another world where everybody becomes angels.

A Present from the Late Father-in-Law

Once a month, a housewife comes to me to consult on her bad condition. One day, when we were having tea after I had flown *ki* energy into her, she started to talk about her concerns about her only daughter.

"She was introduced to prospective marriage partners many times but none goes well. I am really worried about her," she said.

Upon hearing this, I had a vision of a joyful look of her dead father-in-law.

"Your father-in-law says he'd like to give you a present as you were so nice to him when he was alive."

"What kind of present, may I ask?" She looked very happy.

"When you see a black jacket with flowers printed across from shoulders, just buy it. That's his present."

"I understand," she said and left with a confused look on her face. She gave me a call the next day.

"A strange thing happened. A boutique my friend owns had a jacket exactly as you described. I bought it." She sounded very excited.

I was sure that her problem was solved. "Wear the jacket at the next marriage meeting. It'll be successful."

Six months later, as I expected, I had the happy news that her daughter was engaged. At the same time, her health was recovered rapidly as her worries went away.

Solve whatever worries as soon as possible for your physical health.

A Day of the Equinox

In Japan where people who have Buddhism background, we remember the dead and often visit the ancestral grave on the week of equinox. We call equinox "*higan*," and *higan* literally means "another world."

One equinox day, I was invited to my clients' house for consultation. While having a conversation, my client started to speak about her dead father-in-law. Suddenly "*tofu*" came up to my mind, so I asked her,

"It is very strange but I had a vision of *tofu*. Do you know why?"

My client looked so surprised. "My father-in-law hated white rice, so I always had to prepare *tofu,* just for him, everyday," she answered.

"I think your father-in-law asks you to offer tofu instead of rice to his tablet."

"So, the likes and dislikes remain the same even if one has passed away…." My clients said.

The person who passed away barely speaks. When they have messages to someone in this world, they usually show me a vision. That's why I always ask my clients why I have those visions and their interpretations. It is important to listen to the message and try to understand what it really means.

Remembrance of the Dead Son

A mother who lost her son in an accident visited me. She looked gentle. "I think my son wants to say something to me. Could you hear him?"

I had a vision of a photo album and shoes through the clairvoyant power using *hado.*

"I know…it is the photo album filled with the pictures of the *danjiri* festival in *Kishiwada, Osaka.*"

As he grew up in *Kishiwada*, he naturally loved the *danjiri* festival. The *Danjiri* festival was his part of life. He dashed out of the house and showed his valiant figure during the festival. The photo album filled with his memory was very precious for his parents.

I guessed that her dead son looked delightedly at his parents who were joyfully looking at the photo album.

At the mention of shoes, his mother still had regrets that she was so heart-broken that she has forgotten to put his shoes in his casket.

"I think I had the vision of shoes because you worry too much. Bow to the Buddhism altar and ask him the permission to discard the shoes."

The parents now enjoy the *danjiri* festival with their son's friends, inviting them to their house.

It is a very devoted son who cheers up his parents at the time of the festival even after his death because he received so much love and so many good memories from his parents while he was alive.

Even a smallest memory could be the most precious thing for the family.

So Many Good Things and Bad Things

An elderly couple visited me. As soon as my session started, they showed me their daughter's picture and told me;

"My daughter was killed in an accident when she was only 18 years old. Ms. Matsuzaki, can you tell how she feels about her short life? Because she died so young we feel that she might want to do something before her death. If there is something she left behind, we'd like to do it for her so that she can rest in peace."

I flew my *hado* power into the dead daughter. Then I heard her saying,

"Father, mother, don't worry about me. My life was so short but I had done everything before I died. I did so many good things and bad things. I have done everything what I wanted to do."

I explained what I heard to the parents of the dead daughter. Suddenly, they started to cry and told me:

"Ms. Matsuzaki, that's exactly what she said a few days before her death. Now we are sure that she lived her life to her fullest, nothing left behind. Thank you very much."

Their faces became very peaceful.

I have a special gift to hear the message from the people who passed away. In most cases, people who suffered a loss of their loved ones can be healed by understanding those messages from another world.

4. REMOVING THE AGNOY OF DEAD

A Master Carpenter Who Cannot Work

There was a carpenter who had no problems in his daily life but could not move his body at his work. "I heard a lot about you," he said. "Please help me. I am lost because I cannot work."

He has dedicated his life to his profession as a master carpenter. I didn't think he was sick or anything. "I feel that the *hado* power has no effect on you now. Shall I visit your house to investigate the cause of your trouble?" When I am exhausted, another "me" in myself suddenly sniffs danger and refuses to flow the *hado* power in front of clients like him.

A week later, I visited the carpenter's house. As I had anticipated, a dark mood was filled in the air. It happens often. People hardly recognize the stagnant air as they get used to living in the environment.

I sensed that it was not the family but the ancestors who were exhausted. I advised to open up the windows to exchange the stagnant air; then I flew the *hado* power into the ancestors of this family.

The master carpenter started to scream when I was sending the *hado* power.

"Strange…I heard hundreds and thousands chanting the sutras." He said in awe yet with excitement.

I think his ancestors surely received the *hado* power. The master carpenter went back to work next day energetically.

Removing the Agony of the Dead Mother

A single woman in her 30's was living in Sakai-City. She called me and said in a sad voice that she felt that her body was so heavy.

I visited her home. The house was clean and the air was not stagnant. The Buddhist altar was purified and it appeared that she held her ancestors in veneration. I wonder why she was suffering.

She sent me into the living room. While we were making conversation, she suddenly took an ancestral tablet from the altar. I tried to flow the *hado* power into the tablet in front of me. My hand suddenly started shaking.

"I can move my right hand but not my left. Do you know why?" I asked her. She started to cry.

"That's my mother's tablet. She killed herself."

Her mother cared so much about her daughter even after her death. "Don't worry. I will send the *hado* power into her so that she would feel all right."

A few minutes after sending the power, my hand stopped shaking. "Now she feels OK," I told her.

After a little while, her expression started to shine. "Maybe it is just my imagination, but I feel that my body is much lighter."

After this, I kept on flowing the *hado* power into her and carefully observed her movements, which were becoming better and better. She had an easy carriage as though she was dancing.

It is important to understand the thoughts of the dead people and remove their agonies.

A Widow With Neck Pain

A widowed woman in her forties came to see me complaining her terrible neck pain. Even doctors at hospitals hadn't been able to do anything with it. She had a bad complexion. In fact, it was more than bad, it looked eerie. I tried the clairvoyant power with *hado*.

I had a vision. It was a young woman who resembled the widow in front of me. She was ill-treated by her mother-in-law, crawling on the *tatami*

REMOVING THE AGNOY OF DEAD • 21

mats driven by pain. "Do you have someone in your mind?" I asked the widow.

"Yes, my neighbor told me that a woman was ill-treated and killed by her mother-in-law generations ago. I hear that I look very much like her. Of course my family wouldn't tell me anything…."

This kind of thing happened a lot before Meiji Period (mid 19th century). The family held their tongue but her brother-in-law was also killed by a car accident. It was rumored in her neighborhood that there was something in her family, and she had sleepless nights recently.

I tried the clairvoyant power with *hado*, certain that she was haunted by this dead young woman. I guessed that dead young woman wanted the widow of her reflection to know her pain.

I flew *ki* energy into the dead young woman.

All of a sudden, the widow's face brightened. Further, her face transformed into a peaceful expression. She said with a bright smile, "It is strange. My body feels lighter and the pain around my neck has diminished."

I advised her: "Now the pain of the dead woman has been removed. Please serve an extra tea for her on the table when you have one. Offer foods in season at the altar with care.

There are a lot of unbelievable things in the world. Please hold your ancestors in great veneration.

Death in Water

One of my clients asked me to visit their house. I met him in front of a train station and took a taxi to his house. As soon as I had a seat in the taxi, he showed me a picture of a woman, telling me:

"It's my daughter."

I was so shocked because I immediately knew that she was murdered.

"Did she die an unnatural death?" I whispered to him. He nodded silently. After that, we became quiet.

His wife greeted me at the entrance of the house. We all three went into the living room and sat down. The husband showed the picture again and asked me,

"Can you tell us what really happened to her?"

I started to have a vision of water.

"I see water. Was she drawn in water?" I asked the parents of this poor woman.

"Yes. What else can you see?"

"I think what I am seeing is either a lake or ocean. I assume it is an ocean because I see waves" I told them.

"Yes, my daughter's body was found in seashore. She was drawn to death."

I started to have a vision of a ocean surrounded by a foreign landscape, I guess, Southeast Asia. I continued my clairvoyant power.

"I don't know if I should say this…I think that your daughter was killed, and that the murderer hasn't been arrested, is that right?"

The parents nodded with tears and asked me, "Can you see who killed our daughter?"

I saw a man who pushed their daughter from a boat. It was the daughter's husband. I explained to them what I saw.

"I knew it." The father said. I asked him why he said so.

"My daughter appeared in my dream after her death. She said, 'Father, please listen to me. I was killed by my husband. Please believe me.' But I had no way to confirm if my daughter had really appeared in my dream. That's why I asked you to come see me." Father explained.

After his daughter appeared in his dream, he firmly believed his son-in-law had killed his daughter in a foreign land so that he wouldn't get caught.

"He has to pay the price." I told the parents, "Your son-in-law would swell up like a bullfrog's body and die."

"He's already dead, Ms. Matsuzaki," the father told me. "If he were alive, I would do anything to get him arrested… Indeed, he died of pulmonary edema with his lung full of water."

5. FAMILY TIES

Smile of Mountain Cherry Flowers

A mother whose daughter was to take the entrance examination for Music College visited me. "Ms. Matsuzaki, will she pass the exam?" She looked so desperate. Actually, I was personally acquainted with her daughter and I was sure she'd pass the exam because she had good academic ability. Something occurred in my mind.

At that time, I adorned the room with mountain cherry flowers that my friend had given to me. Before replying to her, I put the question to the flowers. I looked at the flower and it was smiling. "Mrs., your daughter will be fine because the flowers are smiling."

She had a graceful manner and always spoke to me with a smile, but she had one bad habit: smoking cigarettes. I always felt uneasy about it, so I advised her. "You should quit smoking, otherwise your graceful manner and gentleness will be completely ruined; furthermore, it may have a negative affect on your daughter's exam."

I don't know if my words made any difference but she quit smoking for her daughter once and for all. Then she dedicated herself to her daughter's education seriously with her natural gentleness, and eventually developed her daughter's gift in music in cooperation with me.

I think the *hado* from the mountain flowers cherry was passed to the mother, and the mother's love was passed to her daughter. The daughter passed the entrance exam with the one of the highest scores.

It is difficult to develop a child's gift solely through taking lessons if they are in a bad environment or have poor upbringing. Sometimes you can solve your problems by changing your lifestyle a little bit.

A Worried Mother

A mother of a student who goes to Osaka University asked for my advice. "Recently I am concerned about my oldest son who lacks energy. I don't know if he worries about his romantic relationship or his friends. Would you send the *hado* power to him?"

I asked her to visualize her son, and then sent clairvoyant power with *hado*. He looked lively from the outside but I saw a dark shadow over his lung. "I am concerned about his lung."

She looked very surprised at first but remembered something. He was a soccer player in high school but she made him quit because his lung exam returned positive.

"He lacks energy because he has lung trouble. I suggest you take him to a doctor."

She thanked me for my advice many times and left in a hurry. "I will take him to the hospital to get exams as soon as possible."

Apparently, her son started to play soccer at the University assuming that his lung was cured. However, he started to notice symptoms and thought "My lung problem has relapsed." He couldn't tell to his mother because he didn't want her to be worried.

Luckily I saw a dark part over his lung with my clairvoyant power, but this was led by his mother's intuition.

A lot of big problems can happen to a family. Those can worsen just because the family members cannot talk about it. In that case, come see me first. It is easier than one thinks.

Sickness of a Boutique Owner

I've known the owner of the biggest boutique in the neighborhood for a long time. Whenever he has a sale in his shop, he calls me and says, "Please flow *ki* energy into me again. For some reasons, I feel secured."

A little while ago, I received a call on my cell phone from the owner. He wanted to ask advice for the period of summer sale. I happened to be near his shop so I visited him directly.

After exchanges of greetings, I felt something strange and touched his shoulder unconsciously as part of a friendship. There was something wrong with him.

"You look different physically. You should go to a hospital with your wife."

Usually, he makes a joke on these things but he didn't say anything this time. It made me feel uneasy.

A week later, his wife called me. "Please come see my husband now. The doctor told us he had a cancer…"

In a hurry I went to their house. Questioning further, they were told that it was the early stage of cancer and could be cured by surgery. "Please flow *hado* power in me for I am worried," he asked.

I flew *hado* energy into the site of his stomach cancer and his shop since my old friend was eager to get back to work.

After that, the operation went well and he recovered in no time. Now he works energetically.

His wife always says to me, "You're something—tell the disease just by touching the shoulder!"

Mother's Pilgrimage

"My mother has a cancer. She looks so down, maybe because of her age. Please flow *ki* into her and make her feel a little better."

I visited the client's house. Her mother was very friendly to me with smiles, and both her posture and behavior looked so graceful. At first glance, she didn't appear to be suffering from cancer at all.

"Oh dear, you look very good," I told her and made her relax, putting my hand on her and trying the clairvoyant power with *hado*. I saw her blood flowing with vigor. I immediately knew that she was recovering. "Your cancer has already been cured. From now on please try to regain your physical strength." I kept on flowing *ki* energy into her.

After a period of time, it appeared that her body became lighter. She started to exercise, stretching her arms and legs and then, "Oh I must visit the restroom," she said, leaving with elastic steps. Her daughter looked very surprised. "I haven't seen her walking that firmly for many years. I am so happy about it."

A month later, the daughter called me again. "The doctor also told me that my mother was recovering. But my concern is that she started to insist to go on a pilgrimage in *Shikoku* for a week."

"Well, I think she shouldn't do it until she is fully recovered…. Anyway, please speak with the doctor and make him decide."

Ultimately, with the doctor's approval, she went on a pilgrimage in *Shikoku* in high sprits but ended up having a relapse, perhaps because she wasn't recovered fully.

In order to keep in shape, it is important for you to be aware of your condition and try to enhance your self-healing ability.

A Boy Who Refuses To Go To School

There was a sixth-grader in elementary school who refused to go to school. Even if he went to school, he returned to home in the middle of the day. His mother came to me for advice.

She told me that his school teacher had said, "As soon as the class starts, he complains of headache and becomes out of control. He cannot concentrate on studying. I asked him and his classmates why, but I cannot find out the reason at all."

The boy told his mother, "I love going to school and I have a lot of friends. No bullying."

I met the boy on a different day. He had returned home in the middle of the day again and it was a pity to see him struggling in such pain. While I watched him, I tried the clairvoyant power with *hado*, and I had a vision of a graveyard. Maybe this was the reason for refusal to go to school. "Mother, is there a graveyard on his way to school?" "Actually yes, there is…." She said thoughtfully.

I guessed that the sense of terror acquired through reading books and telling "scary stories" with his friends lingered in this boy's head and it recurred to his mind when he walked by the graveyard. That experience may act like a haunted ghost and make the brain mechanism go wrong.

First, I flew *hado* power into him to make his mind stronger and instructed him to change his route to school and to take a morning stroll for a while.

After a while, his mother called me with joy, "Thanks to you, my boy is doing all right now. It's as if he is another person. Of course he doesn't suffer the headache during class any more.

This is a common story for children during the growing up ages. If they had the sense of terror more than they can handle, it could cause irrecoverable damage to their brain mechanism. Please keep that in mind.

Domestic Violence I

A woman with exhausted expression came to see me for advice.

"I have a daughter living in Los Angeles. She suffered so much because of her husband's domestic violence…She fears that one day she will get killed. If I were in Los Angeles, I could help her somehow, but I cannot do anything from here. Ms. Matsuzaki, please help my daughter."

I flew my *hado* power into her daughter.

"Your son-in-law is hitting your daughter because he has a fear of losing her. If she tries to escape now, the things could get worse. From now on, I keep sending the *hado* power into your daughter to protect her from the violence. But please give me a little time and be patient. Also keep me posted."

Since then, I have been sending the *hado* power to the woman in Los Angeles. After one month, the mother called me;

"Thank you so much for your help. My daughter says her husbands' violence almost stopped."

I felt so relieved but the daughter still has things to do.

"I am so glad that the domestic violence is stopped. But now your daughter has to file a divorce. I keep sending the *hado* power so that she can get divorced safely. Again, please inform me how it goes."

Another two months passed. I had news from mother that the daughter's divorce was approved and she returned to Japan safely.

Domestic Violence II

A worried mother came to see me for my advice regarding her teenage boy. He has refused to go to junior high school since last year. He shut himself from anybody: he kept himself to his own room and his mother had to leave meals in front of his room every day.

I advised her, "Don't leave the meals in front of his room so that he will eventually come out from his room when he feels hungry. I keep sending the *hado* power into him so that he will regain the strength to go back to school."

I sensed the mother wanted to tell me something else and waited but she didn't reveal her real problems. I just reminded her that she could give me a call whenever she needed me.

One day, I received an urgent phone call from the mother. She sounded panicked.

"Ms. Matsuzaki, Please help me! My son lost control and he is hitting me so badly!"

She was screaming. I immediately understood this was something she couldn't tell me previously. She was too ashamed to tell me that she has been suffering from her son's domestic violence.

I had a vision of the terrifying mother and her raging son in their house. I flew *hado* power into both of them. The mother was still on the phone and told me;

"I cannot believe this…My son suddenly calmed down and went back to his room just now…I didn't know that your power worked so quickly… Thank you so much. I call you back later." She hung up.

Later that day, she called me again;

"I don't know how to thank you. I have been suffering from my son's domestic violence since he refused to go to school. When my son started to hit me earlier today, my husband was home too. He was so surprised and asked me what I have done because my son suddenly calmed down almost the same time I called you. Although my husband has been trying to stop my son's violence for a long time, he hasn't been able to do anything. I told my husband everything; I visited you and asked you for a help. He was not a kind of person who believed in this kind of things, but he had no choice but believe in your power now."

I kept on flowing *hado* power to her son thereafter; soon he started to go back to school. A year later he passed the high school entrance examination and now enjoys his school life.

6. HOUSE PHYSIOGNOMY

Restaurant of a Happily Married Couple

There was a small restaurant run by a married couple. The wife visited me after hearing my reputation. "We lost customers right after the renovation. We have no choice but close the restaurant if the customers don't come back. Please help us."

I didn't think even *hado* power would make any difference in this case. I declined her request in a polite way but she insisted that I come see her restaurant once as she had nothing to lose.

So I went to her restaurant. I felt that the restaurant was very neat and cleanly kept, but that the most important areas such as the cash register, entrance and the table area were dirty and shady. When I entered from the main entrance, the inside appeared very dark.

I sat down at a table and flew the *hado* power into the place. Too many plants and decorative figurines near the entrance blocked the way. "I know you were so conscious of your customers that you put a lot of things at the entrance; however, it backfired and pushed away the customers. I think you should make it simpler. Please consider the minimalist but impressive interiors that make you feel relaxed."

There was another thing. They were overly concerned with their entrance, ignoring the old tables that made the restaurant look odd. I advised them to pay more attention to the old tables and decorate them beautifully.

One month later, the wife called me to tell her thanks.

"According to your advice, our customers came back. We made the entrance simpler and put lovely cloth on the tables. Those are well received. Thank you so much."

Their business came back due to the effect of *hado* power and well-balanced interior décor.

Extension of the House

A master carpenter brought his customer to me. She was in her fifties but she looked much younger. She planned to extend her house and she asked me for my advice on when and how to do the extension because she was very concerned about it.

They took me to the house. While I sent the *hado* power to the site where they expected to build the extension, I had a vision of a man in his sixties, shouting, "*banzai* (means hail or long life)" with delight. I mentioned this to the carpenter and the customer.

"Really,?" she said. "He must be my husband who passed away two years ago. We'd been talking about this house extension, here, to build our new bedroom…"

Now she's living with her son's family. As her grandchildren grew, they started to think about the extension again. She remembered what she used to talk about with her late husband and started to realize that she wanted to make his dream come true. That's why she went to the master carpenter.

"I am very happy to know my husband is glad about the extension. Thank you very much." Her eyes sparkled. She looked somewhat younger than before. I felt the deep ties in this couple and shed tears in sympathy.

She is very fortunate because she lives with her family: the trend in Japan today is that the parents and the sons live separately. She should go ahead with the extension, not only making the dream of the dead husband come true, but also enabling her to live close to her children and grandchildren.

I advised her that when she was ready for another extension, to contact the specialists and make them design the house for a large family. I was very happy to send the *hado* power to a happy family this time.

The Wrath of Fire God

There was an average professional couple. They asked me to examine the house they were planning to buy, as they were a bit worried.

I went to the house accompanied by the couple and their real estate agent. The house was located near a hill in *Hannan* City, Osaka. It was rather small but the façade looked very solid. We all went inside. When we reached the kitchen, I shouted in surprise. I had seen a burst of flame. I became stiff in a short moment. I told everybody to stay quiet and sent the *hado* power to the flame.

Then I had a vision of an unknown married couple who argued every day. I asked the agent, "I think the previous owners had an extremely bad relationship and had terrible quarrels. That's one of the reasons they had to sell their house. The fire god is in wrath."

The agent said, "I am surprised that you could find out that detail."

In spite of all this, the couple really liked the house. "OK, I understand." I told them, "You won't have any problem if I appease the wrath of god. I will send the *hado* power from now."

I have experienced many similar cases. After buying a house, a couple started to quarrel so badly, their children started to have concentration problems, the husband hardly returned home, and so on.

In those cases, I can easily figure out the underlying reason by using my clairvoyant power with *hado* at the location. Please seek for advice as nothing can be solved if you worry by yourself.

Spirits Reside Inside of Things

"I have some office buildings but we don't have enough tenants. Will you flow the *hado* power to buildings so that we have good tenants moving in?"

A business woman in her mid-40's came to see me for help. She took me a place where her buildings were located.

"Will you tell me which one is your building?" I asked her.

"That one, over there." She pointed. I started to flow *hado* power into the building. Something unexpected happened.

"I smell *kimchi* (Korean pickles flavored with garlic), do you know why?" I asked her. She looked so surprised.

"How did you know? I am naturalized Japanese. My grandparents were originally from Korea and I constructed buildings with their estate."

I never even imagined that she was naturalized Japanese. The smell of *kimchi* became stronger and now I smell fish too. I asked her why.

"I think that is the *kimchi* my grandmother made. She was from *Pusan*, a Korean City, and they put fish in *kimchi*."

I kept sending the *hado* power. Suddenly I had a vision of a fat elderly woman with beautiful gray hair showing smile. According to my client, she must be her grandmother from *Pusan*. I guessed she was happy receiving the *hado* power.

After finishing flowing *hado* into the building, my client asked me to flow the *hado* power into another building next to it. While sending the *hado* power, this time I had a vision of an old man with big smile. So I asked her,

"This time I see an elderly man who has a bold spot in the middle of his head. Do you know who he is?"

She answered, "It must be my grandfather."

I guess that my clients' grandparents were having considerable feeling for buildings because their granddaughter started her business with their estate. Sometimes spirit resides inside of the things, and sometimes things have its own heart. That's why we shouldn't treat things roughly. Please keep that in your mind.

7. HEALING THE SICK

Father's Hospitalization

One day I had a visitor whose father was suffering from multiple illnesses.

"Ms. Matsuzaki, I heard a lot about you. My father has been suffering from collagen disease for a long time. Maybe because he has been staying home all day, he became very weak; and started to complain about chest pain lately. He is hospitalized now…Will you flow your *hado* power into him? It is pain to see him suffer so long."

I tried my clairvoyant power to see her father; I sensed that the problem is coming from the clients' house.

"I think I have to visit your house; otherwise, my *hado* power will not be fully effective in this case." I asked the client.

So my client took me to her house. I was overwhelmed by the dark and hazy air inside of the house.

"Please open up all windows and exchange the air NOW." I asked the family.

After the stagnant air was gone, I started to flow my *hado* power into the house.

The father was in the hospital and had no idea that what was happening in his house when I started to flow the *hado* power. However, another patient in the hospital told him that he had a much better complexion. In fact, he recognized that he didn't feel his chest pain or nausea that very day. Further, the shadow on his chest X-ray which had been observed before the hospital admission disappeared after flowing *hado* power several times. Doctor discharged him from the hospital soon.

I heard that now he enjoyed his life in full.

The Destiny of Father

A middle-aged woman came to see me all the way from Hokkaido. "Ms. Matsuzaki, I heard a lot about your healing power. My father is very sick; actually the doctor diagnosed that he is having terminal cancer and he is believed to be within 6 months of death. Could you help him to do anything?"

I used my clairvoyant power to see her father. I saw the total blackness over his stomach.

"Is he suffering from stomach cancer?" I asked.

"Yes…" The client from Hokkaido answered.

Further I tried my clairvoyant power. For some reasons, I felt that I could heal his cancer.

"By flowing my *hado* energy, I think I can ease his pain pretty much and ultimately heal his cancer."

"Is that true? Are you totally sure about that?"

"Yes. However, I think he will pass away anyway for another reason…..
I see his destiny…"

"Well, if you can ease his pain, please flow your *hado* power directly into him as early as possible!"

I started to fly to Hokkaido to visit the client's father at hospital once a week. Everything went all right, and he started to feel lighter and lighter; he was finally discharged from the hospital within six months. By that time, I was assured that his cancer would be healed. I kept on visiting him his home in Hokkaido weekly bases. My client was so happy to see his father regaining his health.

However, suddenly, I had sad news from my client. Her father passed away. She was so angry and telling me that I was a con artist and cheated her and her father. I felt sympathy towards her because she just lost her beloved father after having hope that he might live longer. However, at the same time I was so sure that I healed her father's cancer.

Few weeks later, I received a letter from her lawyer. He says that my clients sued me for a fraud. Also the letter notified me that she had brought her father's body to a University laboratory for autopsy.

Another week passed. Her lawyer called me that the client withdrew her complaint. According to the autopsy, they couldn't find any tumor from his organ. Actually, they only found out that the cause of death was heart attack.

Everyone has their own destiny. I can help my clients to ease their pains; however, you cannot alter your destiny by all means. It is very painful for the family, however, that is the fact of life I found out through my work as a healer.

Mother's Operation

An August night, one of my vocal students visited me. She came to see me about her sick mother because I am an advisor at *Izumisano* Senior Care House. She didn't know anything about my *hado* power.

Her mother needed full-time nursing care; she was too weak to swallow, only able to have fluid food. The doctors told my student that her mother wouldn't survive until October if nothing had been done; thus they scheduled an operation in mid September to make an incision in the lower abdomen to insert a tube to administer nutrients directly.

I explained about the *hado* power, and promised her to flow my power into her mother immediately. As she didn't know nothing about my *hado* power, she looked totally surprised and not convinced at all what I said. Anyway, I sent my *hado* power to her mother after she left my house.

Next morning, I received a call from my student. She said,

"Ms. Matsuzaki, something very unusual happened this morning. My mother was able to swallow the normal food! I wasn't convinced about your *hado* power last night, but thank you so much for whatever you have done to my mother! I have never expected my mother could eat again…"

Shortly after this, the operation was cancelled.

The unknown power really exists in this world. Even if you don't believe in this, or if you don't know that I am sending you the power, you are able to receive it and it really works!

In Lieu of Postscript

Three years ago, in the winter of the year 2000, my only child, Takaori passed away in a traffic accident. He was such a good son ~ so kind to me, his friends and acquaintances, and loved by every one.

It is impossible to imagine the agony of a mother who lost an only child. After the accident, I felt like going mad with grief and suffered so long. I thought, "If I could, I would die instead of him, how I am going to live without him…."

I think he worried seeing me suffering so desperately. One night, he appeared in my dream. He told me, "Mother, please don't worry about me. Work hard on your job to help more people who are in pain. I really love your smile when you listen to your clients."

When I woke up, I saw a chink of light, and at the same time, I saw the letters "*Kokoro no Orion*" (Weaving the Sound of Heart) occurred in my mind. I used the clairvoyant power with *hado,* and had a vision of this small booklet titled "Weaving the Sound of Heart."

I believed that this was a precious gift given by my son, Takaori, and it led me to write this book.

With all my heart, I wrote the examples of advice given to my clients with various kinds of problems. I'd be grateful if this booklet could make any difference in solving your problems.

If you would like to know more about the author, Ms. Matsuzaki, and her *hado* power, please visit her website,
http://www.hadopower.com/index.eg.htm or email to info@hadopower.com

0-595-29819-2